# How Your Body Works

## and How to Create Magnificent Health

Claire Louise Hay

ISBN: 1495378802
ISBN-13: 978-1495378805

# DEDICATION

I dedicate this book to my womb. I'm sorry. I love you. I trust you. Thank you for teaching me.

# CONTENTS

# ACKNOWLEDGMENTS

I have unlimited appreciation for the universe, for everything and everyone in it, for every lesson and experience I have had that has led me to this point of sharing what I have learned.

I am extremely grateful to my body for teaching me, talking to me and helping me to understand the truth in order to share it.

# 1 INTRODUCTION

I am a psychic, which only means that I am more perceptive of energy than most and can verbalise it. And I know that we all have access to the everything, to all knowledge. Putting these two together means that I have telepathic access to not only humans, but to spirits, source, higher selves, aliens, animals, angels, trees, rocks and whatever else you can think of that is in our universe. And my body.

I have used this gift to help myself and others heal themselves and release anything that is standing in the way of them having anything they want in life, such as emotions, beliefs, self-doubt, etc. I have used this gift to answer people's most burning questions about themselves and their lives. I also use this gift to quench my unending questioning nature.

I have enjoyed great health for many years. I never get as much as a cold. I don't even have a doctor. The extent of my body's malaise right now is a sore right elbow and forearm from typing and using my iPhone and iPad too much. A stiff neck from my posture when I sit at my desk. A toenail that grows upwards because I used to wear a toe ring that got caught under the nail pulling it up so far that the nail bed was damaged. Slight lower back pain and tummy bloat and pain when I am on my period.

Right now in this very moment I am only feeling my back ache and tummy ache with my period. Tonight I asked my pain what it was trying to tell me and it told me loud and clear. I cannot believe it took me this long to ask it. I guess I believed society, other women and doctors that this pain is a normal part of being a woman and my menstrual cycle. It is not.

My womb told me that it has been trying to get my attention for a very long time. It has been giving me pain every month of my life since the age of 11. It has been waking me up in the night, in an attempt to make contact with me when I am at my most receptive. But I still didn't listen to it until tonight. For all the time that I have ignored its messages I am very sorry.

You see, I learned to trust and believe in my body years ago. I learned not to trust and believe in doctors and people who view my body as being flawed. It is for this reason that my body hasn't needed to get sick. It didn't need to communicate anything with me because I was at peace with it. I love my body.

But I was missing these few signals from my body that I have just owned up to, I was accepting them as a part of me, as expected, instead of accepting my ultimate wellbeing and wholeness as my truth. I had got caught up in some lies about my body.

This is what my sexual organs told me tonight when I asked them what they are trying to tell me with this pain:

You have never loved and trusted us (they are crying like a wounded child as they say this). We are your ultimate creativity, we are the part of you that has created your three children and you didn't trust us.

You believed that we were a problem right from the moment we made ourselves known to you, instead of the wonderful gift that we are. You believed that we are bad, that sex is bad, that it's bad to get pregnant and that you'd better not get pregnant. You believed that we are bad, that we cannot be trusted to work perfectly for you.

You believed that we were out of control and needed to be brought into your control. You believed that we couldn't be trusted to know when you wanted or didn't want a child, so you were in fear of us and attempted to control us with force. We showed you every time that we didn't need to be controlled, that you could trust us, we showed you that you didn't need any birth control, that we could be trusted, but you didn't listen to us. (I reacted badly to every type of birth control, the pill made me feel depressed, the coil gave me a constant womb infection until it was gone, I was allergic to condoms and the cap. When I used no contraception I was fine, no sexual health problems, no unwanted pregnancies).

You didn't trust us when you were pregnant. We knew what to do but you didn't believe us. You believed a doctor who told you that we cannot be trusted and we must be controlled. You didn't trust us to give birth by ourselves. We tried to let you know. (I had an extremely painful, more than usual, assisted birth with drugs to speed up the contractions

3

so much that I didn't have a break between them, lay flat on my back, terrified)

We wanted you to love and trust us and you distrusted and hated us. We cannot function well without your love and trust. We kept on telling you. (I had womb infections after every pregnancy. I have had an aching lower back and tummy with every period.)

You learned from experience that we would not give you a child when you didn't want a child, but this was still originating in doubt of us, that maybe we can't make babies anymore for you: we can, we always will as long as you might want to have babies.

We showed you that we could, but your mistrust of us was so great that we could not sustain the pregnancy for you (I got pregnant a few years ago and lost it at 8 weeks because of a womb infection).

We cannot function under these conditions. We cannot be the amazing organs that we are and serve you when you feel this way toward us. We want you to love us and trust us. If you love us and trust us then we can work perfectly for you.

Message received loud and clear. I am guilty of everything they have said. I haven't been listening to them, loving them and trusting them. But I am now. (Phew! Safely dodged a menopause full of painful messages there)

I spent the last few hours apologizing to them, loving them and trusting them. Then they told me to write this book.

# 2 YOUR BODY IS…

Your body is not what you have been led to believe it is.

Here is my truth.

YOU are consciousness, not your body. Your body is a projection of that consciousness.

The body is not as real or fixed as we might have been led to believe. We can change our minds in an instant and in that same instant we can change our bodies, too. Our body is like a movie being projected and our mind is the projector. Just like a movie constantly changing depending on the input, so our body constantly changes depending on our input.

Our body changes in every moment depending on our consciousness, what we believe and think.

Before you can create magnificent health you need to understand who you really are and what your body really is.

You are a creator spirit. You are a part of source, the universe, the everything or God. You have all the power of source at your finger tips. You are not just like God, or source, but you are a fragment of source. If you imagine source to be an ocean, you are a droplet in that ocean, part of it, indistinguishable from it, with the same characteristics as it, made of the same stuff – then you are getting somewhat closer to the truth of who you really are.

You have a higher self in spirit form that is all knowing, meaning it has complete access to the everything. Your higher self has access to all knowledge, all energy, everybody, everything and every other higher self. Your higher self is in spirit form all of the time, it is the real you. Your higher self is in spirit form even when you are incarnated on this planet.

The access to everything that I talk of is energetic access. Everything is energy.

Physicality is our perception of all energy other than and including ourselves through the filter of our own energy.

What we see and experience as our reality is the projection of our energy and perception of other energy in relation to ourselves.

What we see and experience as our body is the projection of our energy and perception of our body in relation to ourselves.

**Why do we have this illusion of our physical bodies and why is our higher self doing this to us?**

Our higher selves created an aspect of ourselves to have a human experience.

We gave ourselves a body because we are here in this human experience in order to create things, to have a physical experience of creation. Our higher self already has a spiritual experience of creation on a purely energetic level, but we wanted to try it out physically.

Just as it's not enough to know about a delicious strawberry, we want to taste it. Just as it's not enough to know about sex, we want to do it. Just as it's not enough to know that we could write a book, we want to actually write it. Our higher self wanted to experience creation, too.

We have this drive to experience things in the physical for fun, to experience creation at a deeper level. So we have physical bodies in order to make this possible.

Our physical bodies are created anew in every moment of our lives with our consciousness.

A person with multiple personalities can have completely different bodies dependent on the personality that presides in the moment. One personality can have a physical ailment, while in the next moment that same body with another personality no longer has that ailment. The physical changeover is instant.

We can change our bodies in an instant without multiple personalities if we truly know and believe in our bodies.

However, the large majority of us have grown up in a society full of doctors, scientists and people who do not trust the body. We have learned to trust those people instead of our own bodies and our bodies are screaming at us to be heard.

Your body can be trusted. It knows exactly how to function. It needs very little help to function perfectly.

All your body needs is love, trust and support in the form of nutritious food when it asks for it, movement when it asks for it, water and respect. Respect for your body is not harming it with chemicals, drugs, pollution, trying to control it with food, excess exercise, force, surgery.

Your body believes you when you have a belief about it, it manifests it into being.

I was in Uganda with my 10 year old son and boyfriend at the time, Kenny. We were helping out at an orphanage that one of our friends, Helen, was also working at. When we arrived we sat down with Helen for a meal and she told us how so many people there were getting malaria, she said "It's not a matter of *if* you get it but *when* you get it"

As Kenny was agreeing with Helen on that point, I quickly whisked my young impressionable son away from the table and into our room. I told him "We will not get malaria. We know that people only get malaria when they believe in it. We don't believe in it. We will be fine. They can get malaria if that's what they wish to believe, but we don't need to have that experience." I carried on until I brought him back to his inner knowing of wellbeing. I advised him to say a quiet NO inside if he hears that again and to walk away wishing them well.

Sure enough, about 2 weeks later Helen and Kenny were struck down with malaria. My son got scared, he started to develop the symptoms of malaria, we went to the lab to find out that he didn't have it. Around the same time I had a mosquito bite that was inflamed to the size of an egg, it pulsed bright red. My immune system was fighting something aggressive (I love and trust my immune system). Helen and Kenny recovered and my son and I were not touched by malaria the whole time we were there.

Be careful what you believe, you will manifest it into being. There is no need for you to manifest illness when you can manifest total wellbeing.

Be careful of listening to doctors, scientists and other people. They will give you beliefs that your body cannot be trusted when it can. There is no need for you to manifest problems when you can manifest total wellbeing.

## But isn't it dangerous not to get tested for bad things?

Yes, if you do not love and trust your body. You would be advised to get it checked out because you will be manifesting disease in it right now.

No, if you love and trust your body.

In fact quite the opposite is true if you love and trust your body: it is dangerous to trust someone who is looking for problems in you, because they will manifest problems in whatever they focus on. Don't let their focus be you!

Doctors are trained to look for problems, they are negatively focused on you. They are trained to use drugs to mask the problems they find (or create). They are legal drug pushers, creating the need for their product then distributing it. Some doctors realise this and change their ways, but they are few and far between right now.

Scientists will find whatever they are looking for in their experiment – it's how the universe works. If a scientist is looking for a positive result and has no doubt about themselves, they will get a positive result. If a scientist is looking for a positive result and doubts themselves, they will receive a negative result. If a scientist is looking for a negative result and has no doubt in themselves, they will get a negative result. If a scientist is looking for a negative result and has doubt in themselves, they will get a positive result. Then these scientists share their creations with the world as if they just found it instead of having just created it themselves, "I got what I was putting out" only they don't say it in those words because of their lack of wisdom and so they mislead everyone into thinking they have found truth when they only found a reflection of themselves. Science only ever proves one thing – that the universe works in the way that it does, consistently, you get back what you put out.

It is safe to trust your body.

I have been to a doctor 3 times in the past 13 years. I regretted it every time. I had to recover from the negative beliefs they told me and I believed. My body instantly manifested problems after seeing them. I was not strong enough in my belief in that part of my body, which is why I went to them in the first place. If I had have been strong in my belief in that part of my body I would never have gone to a doctor in the first place. When I trust and love my body, I am healthy and do not need testing for anything.

I listen to my body, I am in tune with it, I feel something the moment it begins and I listen to it's message and deal with it in the moment. I might get the symptoms of a cold for 10 minutes and I give myself a break from working. I might have had a miscarriage in recent years, but that was after I went to see a doctor who told me that there could be problems because of my age and I believed him because I didn't fully trust my reproductive system back then. Notices to get my cervix scraped or my breasts squished and zapped with radiation that *will* harm my body go straight into the recycling bin. I do not need to look for problems in my body. I trust it and it has never let me down.

It is safe for you to trust your body.

# 3 BE A GOOD BOSS

Your body is your loyal team.

Your body parts are your workers on that team.

They will do anything for you when you treat them well, love and support them.

If you don't trust a body part, if you believe a doctor that tells you that it is flawed, if you don't love that body part, it will cause you pain.

If you don't trust an employee, if you believe someone else that tells you that your employee is flawed, if you don't love that employee, they will cause you pain.

If this pain then causes you to have a doctor remove the offending body part, you have sacked the employee when it was your lack of positive attention that caused the problem in the first place. That employee or body part was a victim of the bosses shortcomings.

If this pain causes you to take drugs to try to control it, you are making the situation much worse for the employee to work well for you and they will start to act out in another way, or the other workers will start to act out.

There is nothing you can do to attack or control this employee or body part that will bring you what you really desire. Only love and trust of them will. An apology for all of the abuse will go down well, too.

If you have already removed a body part, the rest of your body will be in fear of also being sacked by their crazy boss.

The remaining ovary will be angry that you killed her sister.

The remaining leg will be terrified that you will sack it, too.

The remaining breast will grieve the loss of their twin.

The remaining teeth will crumble with fear that the wise ones were taken without reason.

The penis will be in trauma from the loss of the foreskin after it had only just created it.

Apologies are called for. Your body needs to know that you are willing to trust it now. Your body needs to know that it can trust you.

Our bodies are crying out to be heard. No amount of mistrust, control, hate and abuse will ever allow it to flourish and reach its potential.

# 4 OUR BODY'S MESSAGES

Now you know that your body wants to be loved and trusted. Your body can also be trusted to give you clear messages about other things, too.

Our bodies are a projection of our consciousness. This means that our bodies can give us clues about what we need to address in our consciousness.

Our bodies tell us when we don't love and trust that part of our body: that is one kind of message.

Our bodies also convey other beliefs and emotional debris that are within our consciousness.

For example, if you had a teacher who would hit you on the knuckles with a ruler when you got things wrong, whenever you believe that you are wrong your knuckles will hurt. Your knuckles will be telling you "There is nothing wrong with you, believe in yourself. You knew that teacher wasn't being true, now you aren't being true to yourself in the same way." If you never heal this belief and feeling that there is something wrong with you, you will likely get arthritic knuckles. Your knuckles would be connected to not believing in yourself.

For example, if you work yourself to the point of exhaustion and then still carry on working, your body will give you a cold to force you to take the break that you need. If you decide to believe the advertisements on television that you can take a drug and keep going, your body part employees will act out in another way until you take that break, getting more and more serious until you listen.

For example, if you got mastitis in your left breast when feeding your child and you have bad feelings toward that same child in later life (judgment, resentment, displeasure) your left breast will let you know about it with pain. That part of your body is connected with that child, so it will let you know. Contact that child, apologise and instantly the pain is gone (this happened to me).

Your body is not only a reflection of your consciousness in the moment, but it is a collection of all of your life experiences.

We all tend to link certain body parts or symptoms with the same emotional problems or incorrect beliefs as each other because we have all grown up in similar societies having similar experiences. Louise L Hay teaches these common connections in her books (no, she's not related, we just have similar names).

But *your* body is a unique pattern of *your* connections and therefore *your* answers can only be found within *yourself.*

For example, most people will get sore shoulders when they are trying to take too much responsibility on. But your shoulders might be linked to the fear and humiliation that you felt when you were shouted at carrying a heavy school bag.

Your story is in your body. Trust it. Believe it.

When you learn to love and trust your body you can then start to listen to it and put those pieces together to find out what it is telling you.

Great questions to ask yourself are:

When was the first time I ever felt this?

What was going on in my life then?

What was going on within me then?

What other times in my life did I feel this?

What was going on within me then?

How does that match what is going on within myself now?

How did I expect this?

What belief do I have that matches this happening?

Who did I believe about this?

Why do I trust them over my own inner knowing?

The trick is to find the beliefs and/or emotions that match the symptom, sensation or pain.

Always start this healing process by asking yourself if you have been loving and trusting that body part because this is by far the most common problem.

Once you find the belief that is connected with the symptom you need to address that belief, that belief will be incorrect, not your higher truth. Find out what is the truth of it, seek help to find that out. (You could join my Be Healing Inner Circle on www.BeHealing.com and I will personally help you) When your belief is replaced with a positive belief, your fear will be gone and your body part will be happy and healthy, even if your doctor still says it's incurable.

Once you find the emotion that is connected with the symptom, you need to express that emotion to heal it. In all likelihood you did not have the skills, knowledge or support to express your emotions and deal with the situation when the emotional damage was first done. But the great news is that you can heal yourself in retrospect. You can express those emotions fully right now using words to describe it, shouting, crying, however that emotion wants to come out of you, let it out so that it can be released. Write it down, speak it to someone trusted who loves you, speak it into your own eyes in a mirror. Investigate it until you have uncovered every part of how you felt and why, so that you can let it go for good. This isn't about dwelling on the negative, or finding someone else to blame, or reliving past trauma, it is about processing it consciously in the way that you would have dealt with it if you had had the skills, knowledge and support to do that at the time.

Be more like a young child when dealing with trauma (before they learn to repress their emotions and reactions to please other). If someone hurts you yell, shout, cry, tell people, tell them they hurt you, let it out, express it and let it go, then carry on playing.

Be more like an animal about it. Ducks will fight, swim away from each other amongst plenty of quacks and then shake it off with their wings and go about being a happy duck again. Cats will smack you with their claws out if they've had enough of you stroking them and then relax again almost immediately afterward.

However, a damaged human will suppress their feelings, not express them and resent you forever for it whilst developing cancer in their body. Needless to say that isn't good for anyone, not even the person who was spared the correct reaction (their feedback so that they could have learned better) to what they said or did.

It's ok to have reactions to things that we don't like. It is good to allow our emotions out. People need to know at the time if they are hurting someone, it's called consequences and it's how we learn, how we grow, how we become better people.

If we do not express our emotions and let them go at the time of feeling them, we push them down and they remain within us, festering away until (hopefully) we decide to heal it once our bodies have told us enough times about it.

Listen to your body. Ask it what it is telling you. You know how to do this. We all have this ability within us. The ability to find out what is really wrong with us is a part of that body that we can trust!

A few weeks ago I noticed a constant underlying noise of anxiety in my body. I asked my body what it's about. In a meditation my mind kept wandering to me putting honey in my chai. I brought my mind back to the meditation over and over until I realised my body was telling me the problem. The problem was sugar. I stopped having honey in my chai and chocolate that day and the anxiety has gone.

Become aware of your body in every moment. Listen to what your body is telling you. Your body wants you to experience magnificent health and wellbeing. It has everything that you need to be able to do that. Everything that you need to do that is already within you.

# 5 YOUR WEIGHT

Your weight is no different than any other aspect of your body. But I am going to talk about it separately because so many people struggle with controlling their weight.

Your weight is a reflection of your consciousness.

Your body wants to be loved and trusted, including your digestive system, your metabolic system, where your body lays down fat, how it burns calories, your muscles and your skin: all of it.

It wants to be loved and trusted.

It does not want nor need to be controlled, not with drugs, surgery, exercise or diets.

Your body knows what it is doing, your weight is reflecting your consciousness.

What are your beliefs about your weight?

That it is out of control?

That it is difficult to control?

That it is something that cannot be trusted?

That everyone has a problem with their weight?

That your weight is in your genes?

That it's your hormones?

That you would have to exercise like an athlete to have your desired weight?

That you would have to restrict what you eat to have your desired weight?

Putting on weight is a natural part of getting older?

What else is in there?

Write them all down, get them out in the open, in the light of your awareness.

They're not true.

Unless you *have* these beliefs: then they will come true for you and everyone else you convince of your belief.

Love your body and weight just as it is. It is the exact reflection of your consciousness at this moment. It is serving you.

You only need 3 beliefs about your weight:

1. I love and trust my body to maintain my ideal weight.

2. When I feel the need to be thin and not take up very much space, it is a reflection of my wanting to diminish myself instead of own my power.

3. When I feel the need to be thin yet am fat, it is a reflection of my fighting within myself, the need to find and own my own truth.

That's it. No more beliefs required. It's that simple.

When you emotionally eat more food than usual, it is because you are struggling to add something to your life.

When you emotionally stop eating as much food as usual, it is because you are struggling to release something from your life.

See these two situations as signs and you will understand the message your body is giving to you.

When you love and trust your body you start listening to it and respecting it.

You might want to add a little exercise each day when you feel like it, you certainly won't want to work out like an athlete (unless you *are* an athlete, of course, and are inspired to reach physical goals, it's what you love and you couldn't imagine being or doing anything else).

You might want to choose foods that make you feel amazing and eliminate foods that are damaging you, because you will feel which foods damage you when you are listening to your body, you certainly won't want to starve yourself or eat one kind of fruit for a week, or take diet pills or have your stomach surgically altered.

Whatever you might want to start or stop doing it will be unique to you. The amount and type of exercise that will be just right for you will be unique to you. The amount and type of food that will be just right for you will be unique to you.

Only you can listen to your own body. Trust yourself. Trust your body.

Love your body and it will work perfectly for you.

Listen to it and it will be your greatest ally and teacher.

I noticed that my body had started to get heavier. I was always around the same weight until I was about 38, then I started to get a little heavier each year. When I noticed it I began to struggle with it. Starting intense exercise programs and not seeing much difference apart from the loss of my beloved morning mediation and quiet time. Trying to eat less made no difference either. I realised that I was fighting my body so I stopped and just loved and accepted it as it was, trusting that my weight must be right for me right now. As soon as I did that I received an offer of a free book from a lady who had just published it. I accepted the generous offer and when it arrived it gave me all the answers I had been looking for. Those answers were right for me, for my body. She wrote about inflammatory foods causing gradual harm to our digestive and immune systems until we reach a point that the body can no longer mask it and it starts to put on weight. She wrote about a simple elimination diet to find out which of the inflammatory foods were affecting me. I found out from following that that I am allergic to dairy and I react to gluten, sugar and corn. My body started to release the weight easily once I had eliminated those foods.

Whenever I find myself stressing and struggling to manifest something in my life, I put on weight. Whenever I find myself stressed out about releasing something from my life I forget to eat and release weight.

I continue to listen to my body carefully with everything that I eat. Occasionally I eat sugar or gluten or cheese knowing what it will do to me, but knowing the consequences I will do it for the pleasure of the food and I forgive myself and help my body to recover once I have done it. I love and respect my body and I know that it can cope and recover easily when I eat something that it doesn't like occasionally.

You can start to listen to your body carefully, too. You can love and trust your body and your weight.

# 6 YOUR SKIN

Your skin is like every other part of your body. But I'd like to talk about your skin because many people have incorrect beliefs about their skin.

Your skin wants to be loved and trusted.

It knows how to contain every other part of you successfully. It knows how to heal itself if you cut or damage it. It knows how to eliminate toxins. It knows how to stay looking gorgeous. It loves the sun and does not have any problem with it.

Your skin needs to be loved and trusted. It knows what it is doing and it can deal with the natural world perfectly.

It cannot work well when it is not being trusted, when it is being controlled, when it is covered in chemicals, when it is poisoned with Botox, when it is covered in something that stops it from breathing.

When you do not trust your skin and abuse it by trying to control it, it will not flourish.

When I moved to Australia 12 years ago I was amazed at the contradictions I witnessed.

Generally people here believed the science that said that we need to use sunscreen to protect our skin because our skin and the sun were somehow put on the wrong planet together, nature went wrong and they cannot be trusted together. You must put these chemicals on your skin to be safe and healthy!

However, the only people I met (and there were many of them) that had experienced skin cancer were those who used sunscreen. Everyone that I met that doesn't and has never used sunscreen has never had skin cancer. With my own eyes and ears I have experienced the exact opposite of what the scientists tell us. I have experienced that loving and trusting your skin prevents skin cancer.

It is not safe to try to control your skin and believe that your skin and the sun cannot be trusted together. It is safe to believe that skin and the sun have been around much longer than you, I and sunscreen and they been living in perfect harmony all that time.

Your skin does not have any problem with nature.

Your skin does have a problem with not being loved, trusted and listened to.

When I started loving, trusting and listening to my skin I stopped using chemicals on it (I was already allergic to sunscreen – thank you skin for saving me!) I started to use only organic food grade products on my skin (that my cats love to lick off me) and I believe that my skin knows how to stay looking amazing.

Some people say, oh be careful of the sun, you'll regret it in your 40's. Then I tell them that I am already over 40 and I don't regret a thing. I look young because I trust my skin and don't abuse it. They think I am a young person who looks old because they don't love and trust their skin.

I love the sun because it makes me feel great and I trust that my body makes me feel great when it feels great. Our skin needs the sun to feel really good, it generates things that the whole body and mind needs beyond what the scientists know about already. The skin loves the sun, trust it, it knows how to deal with the sun.

Sunburn hurts, that is your skin telling you that you were in the sun for too long. No more, no less. Listen to it. It has no need nor wish to punish you for that digression in later life. Just don't spend so long in the sun next time: easy and clear message.

When your skin starts to wrinkle, sag, dim, age, it is because you do not love and believe in it and you aren't listening to it.

I have been blessed with a super-sensitive body that speaks to me in the form of rashes and pain whenever the tiniest bit of harmful substance is put on it. I can tell you that most of the products in the shops that you put on your skin harm me and are harming you. But don't worry, there are alternatives. (Watch my How to be Organic and Toxin-free videos on www.BeHealing.com)

Your skin knows what it is doing. It can be trusted.

Love, trust and listen to your skin.

# 7 YOUR SEXUAL HEALTH

Your sexual health and reproductive system is like every other part of your body. But I'd like to talk about this because many people live in fear of it. It is widely misunderstood even amongst those who are very conscious of their body's truth.

Your reproductive organs are perfectly designed and serve you well.

They are designed not only for child creation but also for pleasure.

They are one of the most amazing and creative parts of us.

They can be trusted to do their job perfectly. Their job is to create children when we want them and to give us pleasure the rest of the time. How perfect is that?

Our reproductive systems know how to make babies, how to grow them, how to give birth to them, how to feed them. How can we not be in complete awe of these amazing parts of us?

However, most of us have grown up in a society that does not believe that our reproductive systems were designed perfectly. We were taught that they are out of control and need to be controlled so that we don't produce baby after baby. We were taught that sex is bad, shameful and wrong. We were taught to be afraid, very afraid, of sexual diseases. We were taught that the body needs help to even fulfill the functions that it does. We were taught that a woman's cycle is her curse and a punishment for being inherently wrong. We were taught that childbirth is not natural and is a medical procedure. We were taught that getting pregnant is bad and shameful unless we have a piece of paper signed by someone who has been appointed to marry people. We have been taught so many lies about our reproductive systems and our reproductive systems are hurting.

Our reproductive systems are a reflection of our consciousness. It reflects what we think and believe.

If we fear sexual disease, we will create sexual disease.

Our reproductive system is designed to make a baby when we want a baby: it's that simple.

But if we fear getting pregnant when we don't want to because we don't love and trust our body, we will create an unwanted pregnancy.

If we fear that our reproductive system is not perfect we will have trouble conceiving.

I used to give Ask Claire readings (and still do on occasion to the members of the Be Healing Inner Circle on www.BeHealing.com) where the customer can ask me any question about themselves and I ask their higher self for the answer. Often the question will be "I am having trouble getting pregnant. Will I have a baby?" Of course, their higher selves answer would be that they can have anything they want. But I would reply "Yes, you will!" and hope that they believe me more than they believe the doctor who is telling them that there are problems. Belief is everything and I am glad to be a positive belief teller. Many babies are here with their rightful parents as a result.

Our reproductive system is designed to be a pleasure organ when we don't want to create a baby.

But if we believe that our sexual pleasure is wrong we will create problems in our body.

Even if we have distrusted our reproductive systems and had beliefs that create sexual disease, we can heal that disease, even when doctors say that it is incurable. Incurable just indicates narrow mindedness and negativity, nothing is incurable.

*"I was in a monogamous relationship and contracted genital herpes from my partner. I was very naïve about sexually transmitted diseases (STD's) so I didn't recognized the early signs of the disease, which for me consisted of blisters showing up periodically on my body. It wasn't until seven years into our relationship that the symptoms progressed and I became extremely ill and got diagnosed with genital herpes. I was devastated beyond belief and hurt because my partner hadn't been honest with me at the onset of our intimate relationship that he had the disease. He even accused me of being unfaithful in the relationship and giving*

*him the disease. Needless to say, this was the beginning of the end of our relationship.*

*According to my gynecologist, genital herpes is incurable so this was something I was going to have to live with the rest of my life and she prescribed Valtrex, an antiviral drug to manage the symptoms when I had an outbreak. I went through a myriad of emotions – anger, shame, grief, depression and didn't share the news with anyone. The episodes of breakouts became more and more frequent due to the stress I was under. I would be bed ridden for several days with each outbreak and found it harder and harder to manage my daily life. Because of the frequency and severity of outbreaks I was having, my doctor suggested going on a daily maintenance program of Valtrex (instead of just during outbreaks) to better manage the disease. This would be the protocol for the rest of my life. This was the final straw for me. There was no way I was going to be on medication for the rest of my life to manage this. There had to be another alternative so I turned to holistic medicine and acupuncture.*

*This was the beginning of me taking control of my life and understanding the disease better and how to manage it by reducing my stress levels. My holistic doctor suggested I read the book "Your Body Speaks Your Mind: Decoding the Emotional, Psychological, and Spiritual Messages that Underlie Illness" by Deb Shapiro. This book changed my life! It taught me how unresolved emotional issues affect your health and even how feelings and thoughts are linked to specific areas of the body along with how to heal your body with your mind. Very powerful stuff. I continued to get stronger and stronger, both physically and emotionally and eventually left the relationship. I've continued on this healing path getting to really know myself and heal myself from my past childhood issues. I've learned firsthand the importance of no longer suppressing my emotions so they don't fester into health issues later on. It's been years now since I've had an outbreak of herpes and deep down inside I had a knowing that the disease no longer lived in my body even though the doctors say it's incurable. I decided to have a blood test done this past year and the results confirmed my knowing. I tested negative for herpes. I had healed myself from this so-called incurable disease.*

*We are so much more powerful than we are led to believe and I now know anything is possible. Don't let anyone tell you otherwise!"*

Susan Schremp
www.InnerPathToHealing.com

You can trust your reproductive system. You do not need to use contraception, you body knows how to respond to your wishes. You do not need to use barriers to prevent sexual disease as long as you don't believe in them in the first place and aren't creating them with your shame of your sexuality. You do not need help in getting pregnant, apart from the obvious. Your reproductive system can keep making babies at any age, it reflects your consciousness, believe it, want more babies at any age and you will get them. Your reproductive system does not need help in order to grow a baby, it knows exactly what it is doing. Your reproductive system does not need help in birthing a baby, it knows exactly what it is doing. Your breasts do not need help in feeding your child, they know what they are doing and they can all do it if you love and trust them!

There is a magnificence about our reproductive systems that the majority of the world has not yet embraced.

There is so much stigma, unhealthy belief, judgment, control, violence and fear surrounding our reproductive organs and sexuality and these are in desperate need of healing so that we can enjoy one of the best parts of our amazing bodies.

The negative beliefs are so ingrained, the fear runs so deep in our society that you might still have your reservations.

All I can do is reassure you from my experience. Once I stopped distrusting my body and stopped using contraception I was very sexually active, with multiple partners, for 8 years. I did not once get pregnant nor contract a sexual disease.

In the last 5 years I have been monogamous and madly in love with a man who was told by doctors that he would never have children because of the poison they pumped him with to kill his childhood cancer. He believed them and never got anyone pregnant in his life, until we got pregnant together. We both wanted a baby and our bodies knew how to make one. Unfortunately, we went to see a doctor, who told us how risky this was at our age with his history and the likelihood would be that there would be something wrong with the baby or we would lose it. We were not strong enough in our belief to counter that negative attack on our bodies and beliefs. We lost the baby at 8 weeks and are grateful for the experience as it brought us closer. We were parents together. We cried together. We shared the experience with each other. We were blessed. We don't regret not having a child together, the desire to have one faded away as we focused on creating other things in the world together. We have bigger babies called our businesses and books that will help change the world to create. (See his work here www.JarrodKnight.com)

My body can be trusted. Your body can be trusted. Behold the magnificence of your reproductive system, because it is truly magnificent and yes, you are in control of it, you always were.

# 8 WHAT IS JUST PHYSICAL?

Nothing.

Nothing is just physical.

Bacteria, viruses, all the reasons you have been led to believe are the *cause* of diseases are just *how* the disease takes you, not *why*.

Nothing is just physical.

Everything in your life experience, including your body, is a reflection of your consciousness.

## But what about hereditary conditions?

Families teach each other their beliefs. It is the beliefs that are hereditary, they are taught and the corresponding symptom or illness goes with it.

Families pass on their emotional issues to each other. It is the emotional issues that are hereditary, they are taught and the corresponding symptom or illness goes with it.

Families pass on their disbelief in their bodies and their belief in the families hereditary condition. This is taught and the symptom or illness will manifest from that belief.

## But what about clusters of cancer in one place?

We each hang out with people who are reflections of us. Everything in our experience is a reflection of ourselves. So a resentful person will hang out with resentful people, live in an area with other resentful people and manifest the same kinds of diseases as a result. They will all manifest the exact conditions around them that they need (the how) to manifest those diseases, whether it is pollution, bacteria, viruses, radiation, however the body can manifest it, it will, in the easiest way possible.

Once one person gets a disease everyone else around them who doesn't love and trust their body will come down with it, because they believe the diseased person and they doubt their body.

## But what about accidents?

There are no accidents. Everything that happens to you is a reflection of your consciousness. Believe you are clumsy and you will be. Don't be in the present moment when you are chopping carrots and you will chop your finger. Don't listen to how you feel about your job and how you really need to leave and do something else instead and you will have a car crash. Believe that the universe and world doesn't support you and you will have back pain or break your back. Keep complaining about things and you will stub your toe. Resent where you came from or your last job and a car will smash into the back of yours.

Everything that you experience is a reflection of your consciousness in that moment.

The bigger the "accident" the more signs you have already ignored instead of listening to your body and to your life.

## But what about children who get sick?

Their experience is a reflection of their consciousness, too.

If it is from birth they came into their body manifesting a challenge, illness or problem, their higher self consciousness created it to benefit them, to help them to grow as a creator spirit.

If it develops in early childhood, they have learned from the people around them that they cannot love or trust their body.

If it develops in later childhood, they have learned damaging beliefs about themselves and learned the emotional suppression that causes these problems.

There is no need to feel guilty about this if you are a parent who fears that you taught your child damaging beliefs and emotional suppression. We are all in this together. We can all heal it together. It's never too late. None of us are to blame, however, we are all responsible for healing this within ourselves and helping those around us do the same.

## But what about when a virus is going around?

If you believe that viruses are the cause of illness, rather than just the way in which your body can give you an illness, then you well get sick every time it comes around.

If you believe that the illness will last 2 weeks because that's how long it lasted in the first person, then you will be sick for 2 weeks. You could believe that it would last 2 minutes and it would. You could believe in total wellbeing and love and trust your immune system instead and you would have no need to get sick at all.

People's beliefs create these epidemics. Epidemics show us the level of consciousness in our society about our bodies and illness.

We could have a wellbeing epidemic if this message gets out!

# 9 LOVE AND TRUST YOUR BODY

Love and trust your body.

Love and trust your weight.

Love and trust your balance.

Love and trust your skin.

Love and trust your toes.

Love and trust your ankles.

Love and trust your legs.

Love and trust your knees.

Love and trust your hips.

Love and trust your torso.

Love and trust your fingers.

Love and trust your hands.

Love and trust your wrists.

Love and trust your arms.

Love and trust your elbows.

Love and trust your shoulders.

Love and trust your neck.

Love and trust your back.

Love and trust your head.

Love and trust your brain.

Love and trust your eyes.

Love and trust your ears.

Love and trust your nose.

Love and trust your mouth.

Love and trust your teeth.

Love and trust your face.

Love and trust your hair.

Love and trust your hair colour.

Love and trust your jaw.

Love and trust your hormones.

Love and trust your heart.

Love and trust your throat.

Love and trust your lungs.

Love and trust your liver.

Love and trust your kidneys.

Love and trust your digestive system.

Love and trust your stomach.

Love and trust your appendix.

Love and trust your intestines.

Love and trust your bowels.

Love and trust your pancreas.

Love and trust your bladder.

Love and trust your prostate.

Love and trust your ovaries.

Love and trust your womb.

Love and trust your reproductive system.

Love and trust your vagina.

Love and trust your penis.

Love and trust your pelvic floor.

Love and trust your weight.

Love and trust your muscles.

Love and trust your tonsils.

Love and trust your breasts.

Love and trust your bones.

Love and trust your joints.

Love and trust your immune system.

Love and trust your lymphatic system.

Love and trust your cardiovascular system.

Love and trust your urinary system.

Love and trust your respiratory system.

Love and trust your nervous system.

Love and trust your endocrine system.

Love and trust your emotions.

Love and trust your feelings.

Love and trust yourself.

Love and trust that inner voice.

Your body will serve you to the extent that you will love, trust and listen to it. You can have perfect health right now.

There are no limitations. There is no limit to how good your body can feel, how you can feel.

There are no limitations. Everybody can have magnificent health, no exceptions.

Create a magnificent body by believing in it.

Create magnificent health by loving, trusting and listening to your body.

Delight in this knowledge that this book has given you. Share it with those you love. Use it to create the wellbeing that you would really like to experience and enjoy it!

# More titles
# by Claire Louise Hay

How to Manifest Money & Live a Magnificent Life

How the Universe Works and How to Create a
Magnificent Life

The Healing Path Within

Beyond 2012: The Ascension Process

The Little Life Coach

The Little Relationship Coach

# ABOUT THE AUTHOR

Claire Louise Hay is the founder of Be Healing and The Business Re-evolution. She is passionate about inspiring and helping others to change the world.

You can find more of Claire's work on www.BeHealing.com to join her Inner Circle for access to all of her programs, guidebooks, meditations, support group and to access Claire's 1:1 support.

You can access Claire's business and life changing program for business owners on www.businessreevolution.com